CONTENTS

DESCRIPTION

Miso is a Japanese word that means "fermented beans." Miso is usually found in the form of a thick paste, and the beans used during fermentation are almost always soybeans. During the soybean fermentation process, grains like barley, rice, or buckwheat might be added to achieve a certain flavor or other desired attribute, but in most situations, soybeans serve as the basis for miso fermentation. (This basic role of soybeans in preparation of miso can sometimes be overlooked because many varieties of miso may take on the name of their added ingredients, like "barley miso" or "rice miso." Yet virtually all of these miso varieties will contain soybeans as a basic ingredient.)

It's worth noting that under some circumstances, you might hear the word "miso" being used to refer to fermentation of a food other than soybeans. A good example is "fish miso." In this case, the term "miso" is being used to refer to the process of fermentation rather than the food being fermented. "Fish miso" is a term used to describe fish that has been fermented using the same basic fermentation process that can be used to produce soy miso, barley miso, or rice miso.

This use of the word "miso" in relationship to fish is important, because it tells us something very special about the miso fermentation process. For many miso eaters, the magic of miso lies in the micro-organism used for its fermentation: Aspergillus oryzae. This micro-organism is a particular type of fungus (a filamentous fungus, also called a "mold") that plays a special role in Japanese and other Asian cuisines. Long before scientists had developed ways of identifying and naming fungi like Aspergillus, cultures in China and Japan had developed special methods of fermenting soybeans (and other foods) that were practical and could be reproduced (assuring that the same mold was used, even though this mold was not yet scientifically identified). "Koji" was the term used to describe the end result when foods were fermented in this special way.

When scientists eventually discovered that the Aspergillus fungus was the key micro-organism involved with koji fermentation, the word "koji" took on a second meaning. While remaining the name for the end-stage product, it also became the name for the Aspergillus fungus itself. Therefore, you can now hear the word "koji" being used to refer to end-products of Aspergillus fermentation like miso or sake or soy sauce, as well as to the Aspergillus mold itself. You can also hear the word "koji" being used to refer to a grain-based starter that is used in the production of the above foods (including soy miso). When "koji" is used to refer to this starter, Aspergillus mold has usually been added to rice that has been pre-soaked and pre-cooked. The result is of this Aspergillus-fermented rice is called "koji." For a second stage fermentation into miso, "koji" starter is then added to soybeans that have also been soaked and cooked, and the entire mixture is allowed to age and ferment into miso. As you can see, the word "koji" can take on a variety of meanings. But these different meanings tell us something important about miso, namely, the special role played by the Aspergillus fungus in its fermentation.

The texture of miso is usually paste-like and relatively thick, along the lines of peanut butter. But the color and taste can vary widely, depending on many fermentation-related factors. In terms of color, the lightest color miso is usually white or beige. This lighter color is often due to inclusion of a large amount of white rice during the fermentation process. When the word "koji" is used to refer to a miso starter made from rice and Aspergillus, white miso is also sometimes described as containing a large amount of koji. (If the koji has been made from Aspergillus fermentation of roasted rice flour, it may become light brown in color, but is often still included in the category of white miso.)

Other names you might hear for different varieties of miso include:

genmai miso (brown rice-containing miso)
soba miso or sobamugi miso (buckwheat-containing miso)

taima miso (hemp seed-containing miso)

natto miso (chutney-type miso that usually containing barley and ginger)

In China, miso is usually referred to as "taucheo," "dajiang," "doujiang" or just "jiang." In Korea, miso may be referred to as "jang" or "dwenjang." In Indonesia it is called "tautjo" or "tauco."

Given this rich history of miso varieties and names across Asia, the Codex Coordinating Committee for Asia (CCA-SIA, part of the Food and Agriculture Organization/World Health Organization of the United Nations) has actually set food quality standards for fermented soy paste that include fermentation by naturally-occurring or cultivated micro-organisms and other production factors. While the United States is a member of the Codex Commission that works to help develop international food standards, we're not aware of any commercially available miso products in the U.S. that show compliance with CCASIA standards on their labeling. Still, we are glad to see attention being paid by an international organization to the quality of this unique and much-loved fermented food.

WHAT EXACTLY IS MISO?

Miso is a Japanese condiment that originally came from China. Doujiang, the Chinese predecessor to miso, was invented as a way to preserve soybeans. The plant was an important crop for replenishing soil, but the beans spoil quickly. The Chinese turned to fermentation to preserve the beans and keep them edible. The Japanese took that idea and made it an art form.

Miso is made from a mash of cooked soybeans and grains (usually rice or barley) mixed with salt and a fungus called Aspergillus oryzae, or koji in Japanese. This mixture is left to ferment in crocks anywhere from a few weeks to over a year. It may be pasteurized, which extends its shelf life but kills some of the enzymes that make miso so nutritious. After that, it's packed in bags and jars, and distributed to markets. It's generally kept in the refrigerator, where it can last a very long time. Even after it's opened, a container of miso can last up to a year covered in the refrigerator.

WHAT DOES MISO TASTE LIKE?

There are many types of miso. Depending on how long it's aged, the type of grain, and the proportions of the ingredients, the flavor can be sweet or salty, mild or pungent. The variety can be a bit confusing, but it's easier to navigate than the worlds of cheese or wine. Start just by looking at the color of the miso, which is a good indicator of how strong it will be. There are two broad categories: light and dark. In North America, the most common misos are made with white rice (this is called kome), so that's what you're buying unless the package states otherwise.

Light misos (shiro, in Japanese) are mild and slightly sweet. In general, these white and light yellow misos have less salt and more koji. That speeds up fermentation, so this type of miso is aged less for a sweet, lightly fermented flavor.

Dark red and brown misos (aka) have deeper flavor. This category is made with more salt, which allows for longer fermentation times—generally one to three years—and the development of complex, umami-rich flavor with a bit of funk. In addition to the most common red aka miso that's made with white rice, it's generally easy to find brown rice miso, called genmai in Japanese, which is an earthier alternative.

HOW IS MISO USED?

This thick paste packs a lot of flavor, so a little goes a long way. The only time you would use it on its own is as a rub for meat or poultry, where it acts like an exceptionally flavorful marinade and is rinsed or wiped off before cooking. More often, it's combined with other ingredients to balance its potent flavor. Miso can be simmered in soups, stews, or braise just be sure to dissolve it in a bit of hot liquid before adding it to the pot so that it doesn't sink to the bottom and burn. It can also be used raw, whisked into vinaigrettes, sauces, and dips.

There's as much versatility in pairing misos with other foods as there is in how to use them. On the following pages, I've shared some of my favorite ways to use the more common types: White miso enlivens the vinaigrette for a fall salad of beets, apples, and bitter greens; red miso combines with kombu dashi to become a deeply flavored broth for a satisfying vegetarian sweet potato and kale soup; and brown rice miso makes duck legs succulent and savory. These recipes are sure to start you on a long-term love affair with miso, as I've had.

INDIVIDUAL CONCERNS

Miso and Food Allergies

Soybeans and the foods made from them, including miso, are among the eight food types considered to be major food allergens in the U.S., requiring identification on food labels. For helpful information about this topic, please see our article, An Overview of Adverse Food Reactions

In addition to the general allergy-related issues described above for soybean-containing foods, there is some research information specific to miso that is important to consider. First is the issue of protein P34. In some studies, this protein has been found to be one of the primary allergenic proteins in soy. However, at least one study on consumption of Korean miso has shown an undetectable level of protein P34 (with a detection level of 0.45 nanograms) in the miso, making fermented soybean paste a potentially less antigenic (allergy-causing) food than other forms of soy. This potentially reduced allergy risk from miso versus other soy foods makes sense to us. The fermentation process—especially over a period of time involving months or years—is likely to result in substantial modification of the proteins in soy, including potentially allergy-causing proteins like P34.

Some of the anti-cancer benefits of soy miso might

be related to its potential strengthening of the immune system. (Weakened immune system function is a risk factor for many types of cancer.) Research studies show that during the soy miso fermentation process, there is significant potential for the creation of immuno-supportive substances. For example, we've seen a study in which soybeans fermented with the help of the bacterium Tetragenococcus halophilus showed the ability to increase T helper type immunity. Since immune system function often depends on a unique set of peptides (protein building blocks), transformation of soy proteins during fermentation is likely to provide the immune system with some helpful peptidesand eventually lowering our risk of cancer through added immune system support.

Miso and Thyroid Health

Along with the increasing presence of soy foods (such as miso) in grocery stores and on restaurant menus has come increasing controversy over soybeans and thyroid health. We're not surprised to find strong conflicting opinions in this area because scientific research on thyroid and soy is both complicated and inconclusive.

Miso and Acrylamide

When certain foods are cooked, their amino acids (protein building blocks) can interact with their simple sugars to form acrylamide. Acrylamide is a potentially toxic and potentially cancer-causing substance that can be naturally present in uncooked, raw foods in very small amounts, but can be formed in much large quantities in certain cooked foods. Grain-based coffee substitutes and fried potato chips are examples of foods that can contain high amounts of acrylamide. Even though you may find some websites listing miso as a high acrylamide food, we have not found any indexed journal research studies to support this finding. In fact, we have seen several studies on a related soy food - soy sauce - showing no detectable levels of acrylamide. The absence of high acrylamide levels in soy miso makes sense to us, because traditionally prepared soy miso does not undergo any high-heat processing, and also because the sugar content of miso is relatively low when soybeans make up the bulk of the miso ingredients. (Cooked soybeans contain only 2-3 grams of per half cup of total sugars.) In addition, traditionally fermented miso should definitely not be classified as a processed food that is comparable to potato chips or a grain-based coffee substitute. It is a natural food based on whole soybeans and natural processing of these who soybeans by micro-organisms.

Infants and Miso

One study from Japan has shown that breast-fed infants already diagnosed with atopic dermatitis (an inflammatory skin condition) experienced a worsening of dermatitis symptoms when their mothers consumed miso soup and soy sauce. However, the result here does remind us of the importance of considering food sensitivity in the feeding of infants, and the potential difference between individual concerns for infants versus adults involving soy foods, including miso.

Nutritional Profile

Miso is now known to contain phytonutrient antioxidants including phenolic acids like ferulic, coumaric, syringic, vanillic, and kojic acid. Particularly interesting are new additions to the list of miso antioxidants that are related to its fermentation. In several recent studies, the amount of certain antioxidants in miso appears to increase when fermentation is carried out for a longer period of time. For example, several DDPH (2,2,-diphenyl-1-picrylhydrazyl) antioxidants that can help scavenge free radicals in the body have been shown to increase in number as the length of soy miso fermentation time increases.

Miso is a very good source of copper manganese and a good source of vitamin K, protein, zinc, phosphorus, dietary fiber and omega-3 fatty acids.

HEALTH BENEFITS OF MISO

Here are some health benefits offered by Miso:
Offer probiotics

As Miso is fermented, it contains live active cultures which acts like a yogurt in digestive system. Fermented miso is an excellent source of beneficial probiotics with no dairy for those with lactose or dairy sensitivities to foods such as yogurt, kefir and cultured cheeses. Fermented foods contain probiotic bacteria which thrive in our gut microbiota by increasing immunity and promoting digestion. Probiotics helps to promote immune function, enhance digestion, better cognitive health, and reduce the chances of allergies, mood regulation, lower chances for obesity and appetite control.

Assist digestion

Miso soup is a healthiest way to promote digestion. Miso contains beneficial probiotics which combats digestive problems that caused an imbalance in gut bacteria such as diarrhea, constipation, bloating, gas and IBS. Probiotics is helpful for those people who are suffering from serious problems such as candida viruses, food allergies, leaky gut syndrome and ulcerative colitis. Probiotics cleanse the system and is known to speed up the ability of the body to heal gut associated illnesses.

Prevention of high blood pressure

Though Miso has high content of salt, it is associated with prevention of hypertension according to both experimental and epidemiological evidence. Researchers believed that sodium found in Miso acts differently in comparison to sodium chloride alone. The biological effects may be caused due to longer fermentation periods of soybeans, rice grains and barley grains above 180 days. The conducted study shows that rats with systolic blood pressure that received 2.3 percent of sodium chloride was increased significantly but the rats who receive same amount of salt from Miso do not experienced these effects. Despite the intake of sodium increased, the blood pressure of rats did not increased when fed diet of miso.

Cancer prevention

Miso contains immune promoting probiotics, antioxidants and vitamins which includes coumaric, feruic, phenolic acids, vanillic, syringic and kojic acid which is associates to prevention of cancer. As miso is fermented for many months or years, its antioxidant content seems to improve. Miso is helpful for preventing radiation injury and progression of cancerous tumor. Researchers exposed that Miso having longer fermentation time promote healthy cell survival in mice by following radiation treatment and also prevent tumor growth. Fermented miso shows the inhibition of cancerous colon cells development in mice. Miso helps to effectively neutralize free radicals and suppress mammary cancer tumors such as breast tumors, lung tumors and liver tumors in mice. The fermentation process for prolonged time period is vital for protecting cancer and radiation effects.

Great source of nutrients

Miso is a probiotic food which activates certain enzymes found in grains and beans that allows better absorption of nutrients such as manganese, copper, vitamin K, vitamin B and phosphorus. Soybeans when fermented include various phytochemicals such as isoflavones, vegetable fiber, melanoidin and saponin. Miso is a great source of plant based protein which provides two grams in a serving of one tablespoon.

Cure for hangover

Body requires water, amino acids, minerals and vitamins for flushing out alcohol from a system after a night of drinking. Miso soup contains all these things along with sodium which helps to rehydrate.

TYPES OF MISO

Most of the people are familiar with dark brown coloured miso but in fact there are many variations of Miso, each with a difference in base ingredients, cooking methodology and fermentation times.

Kome miso:
Also known as rice miso, it could be yellow, red, yellowish white etc. Reddish miso is prepared from steamed soybeans. Whitish miso is made from boiled soybeans. In Hokuriku and Kinki areas, Kome miso is consumed more.

Mugi miso:
Also called barley miso, it is a whitish miso which is produced in Western Chugoku, Kyushu, and Shikoku areas. In the northern Kanto area, another reddish mugi miso is produced which possess a peculiar smell.

Mame miso:
Soybean miso is a darker, more reddish brown in comparison to kome miso. It is not sweet as other varieties but has astringency and good umami. It needs a long maturing term. Mostly, it is consumed in Aichi prefecture, part of Mie prefecture and part of Gifu prefecture. Soybean miso is also known as hatchō miso which has its origins during the Sengoku era in Mikawa Province. The processing method remains unchanged with large wooden barrels and stones on the lid.

Chougou:

Awase miso or mixed miso comes in various types as it is a combination or compound of other varieties of Miso. It promotes the weak points of each type of Miso.

Akamiso:

Red miso is aged for more than one year. The color gradually changes from white to red or black due to the Maillard reaction. It has saltiness flavor with some astringency with umami. It is a stronger-tasting miso.

Shiromiso:

White miso has rice, barley and a small quantity of soybeans as its main ingredients. Miso would be red or brown if greater quantity of soybeans is added. White miso has a very short fermentation time in comparison with red miso. The taste is sweet and umami is soft or light.

MISO SOUP RECIPES

A Japanese-inspired take on traditional chicken noodle soup. Full of fresh ingredients and delicious flavor!

Prep: 35 mins

Cook: 22 mins

Additional: 10 mins

Total: 1 hr 7 mins

Ingredients

1 tablespoon grapeseed oil, or more to taste

5 carrots, chopped

2 eaches leeks, diced

5 ounces shiitake mushrooms, sliced

1 onion, diced

2 pounds skinless, boneless chicken thighs

1 pinch salt and ground black pepper to taste

8 cups chicken broth

½ cup miso paste

8 cloves garlic, minced

1 tablespoon soy sauce

1 (2 inch) piece ginger root, grated

1 dash sriracha sauce, or to taste

½ head napa cabbage, torn into pieces

1 head baby bok choy

Directions

Step 1

Pour grapeseed oil into an electric pressure cooker (such as Instant Pot®). Add carrots, leeks, shiitake mushrooms, and onion; cook and stir on the Saute setting until softened, about 5 minutes.

Step 2

Season chicken thighs with salt and pepper; add to the cooker. Pour in chicken broth. Seal and cook on the Soup setting for 7 minutes. Release pressure naturally for 10 minutes according to manufacturer's instructions. Cover the vent with a dishtowel and release remaining pressure with the quick-release method.

STEP 3

Remove chicken thighs and shred with 2 forks on a cutting board. Return to the cooker with the miso paste, garlic, soy sauce, ginger, and sriracha sauce. Cook and stir on the Saute setting until miso paste dissolves, about 5 minutes. Stir in cabbage and bok choy pieces; cook until softened, about 5 minutes.

Cook's Note:
You can add rice noodles if desired. If using, add them to the pot once the liquid comes to a boil and cook as directed on the package.

Nutrition Facts
Per Serving:

270.1 calories; 24.3 g protein; 17.4 g carbohydrates; 74.5 mg cholesterol; 2047.2 mg sodium.

Authentic Miso Soup
Made with kombu, bonito flakes, and miso paste, Japanese miso soup is a simple and comforting.

Prep: 15 mins

Cook: 15 mins

Total: 30 mins

Ingredients

4 cups water

1 (4 inch) piece dashi kombu (dried kelp)

½ cup bonito flakes

½ (12 ounce) package tofu, cut into chunks

1 teaspoon dried wakame

3 tablespoons miso paste

¼ cup chopped green onions

Directions

Step 1

Heat water in a large pot over low heat. Add kombu and cook until the mixture just begins to simmer. Stir in bonito flakes until combined. Remove pot from the heat and let dashi sit, uncovered, for 5 minutes. Strain and set aside.

Step 2

Heat 3 1/2 cups dashi in a pot over medium heat. Add tofu and wakame; stir to combine. Remove 1 cup warmed dashi to a small bowl and whisk in miso paste. Pour miso mixture back into the pot with remaining dashi. Stir until warmed through. Serve garnished with chopped green onions.

Per Serving:

64.9 calories; 6.2 g protein; 4.9 g carbohydrates; 0 mg cholesterol; 510.9 mg sodium.

Miso Soup with Shiitake Mushrooms

A delicious Japanese soup with mushrooms and tofu.

Prep: 10 mins

Cook: 10 mins

Total: 20 mins

Ingredients

4 cups vegetable broth

4 shiitake mushrooms, thinly sliced

¼ cup miso paste

4 teaspoons soy sauce

⅓ cup diced firm tofu

2 eaches green onions, trimmed and thinly sliced

Directions

Step 1

Bring the vegetable broth to a boil in a saucepan. Add the mushrooms, reduce heat to low, and simmer 4 minutes. Stir the miso paste and soy sauce together in a small bowl; add to the broth along with the tofu and continue cooking for 1 minute more. Pour the soup into bowls and top with the green onions to serve.

Per Serving:
91.6 calories; 5.5 g protein; 11.8 g carbohydrates; 0 mg cholesterol; 1405.9 mg sodium.

Pumpkin and Tofu Miso Soup
A delicious Japanese-style miso soup suitable for vegetarians and vegans.

Prep: 15 mins

Cook: 15 mins

Total: 30 mins

Ingredients

¼ small pumpkin - peeled, seeded, and cubed

1 (2 inch) piece fresh ginger, cut into matchsticks

2 tablespoons soy sauce

2 ounces buckwheat noodles

3 ½ ounces firm tofu, cubed

2 teaspoons miso paste

2 teaspoons sesame oil

2 eaches green onions, finely chopped on the diagonal

2 large red chile peppers, sliced on the diagonal

2 tablespoons toasted sesame seeds

2 tablespoons chopped fresh cilantro, or more to taste

2 tablespoons pickled ginger

Add All Ingredients To Shopping List

Directions

STEP 1

Bring a large saucepan of water to a boil; add pumpkin, ginger, and soy sauce. Cook pumpkin mixture for about 3 minutes. Add noodles to pumpkin mixture and cook until noodles are slightly cooked, about 4 minutes.

STEP 2

Stir tofu into pumpkin-noodle mixture and cook until pumpkin and noodles are almost tender, 5 to 10 more minutes.

STEP 3

Place 1 teaspoon miso paste into each serving bowl. Ladle cooking water into each bowl and whisk until miso is dissolved.

STEP 4

Divide pumpkin-tofu soup between the 2 serving bowls; garnish each with 1 teaspoon sesame oil, 1 chopped green onion, 1 sliced red chile pepper, 1 tablespoon sesame seeds, 1 tablespoon cilantro, and 1 tablespoon pickled ginger.

Per Serving:

316.8 calories; 12 g protein; 40.9 g carbohydrates; 0 mg cholesterol; 1230.8 mg sodium.

Vegetarian Nori Miso

I began trying to make a clear soup recipe, which quickly grew out of control to incorporate elements of miso, egg drop soup, and seaweed. I serve it as a main dish with a side of brown basmati rice.

Recipe Summary

Prep: 15 mins

Cook: 1 hr 10 mins

Total: 1 hr 25 mins

Ingredients

2 (32 fluid ounce) containers vegetable broth

32 fluid ounces water

2 egg whites

1 ½ cups miso paste

2 tablespoons ginger paste

1 tablespoon sesame oil

2 cups edamame (green soybeans)

2 cups shiitake mushrooms, thinly sliced

⅔ cup chopped spring onions

1 clove garlic, minced

1 teaspoon soy sauce

1 ½ cups cubed firm tofu

1 teaspoon cayenne pepper

⅔ cup crumbled dried nori (seaweed)

2 tablespoons white sugar

Directions

Step 1

Combine vegetable broth and water in a large pot; bring to a boil. Drop egg whites into the boiling broth and boil until egg whites are cooked, about 10 seconds. Skim egg whites from surface of broth using a slotted spoon and transfer to a plate to cool.

Step 2

Reduce heat to medium. Mix miso paste, ginger paste, and sesame oil into broth using a potato masher or ladle until fully incorporated. Add edamame, mushrooms, spring onion, garlic, and soy sauce to miso broth; cover pot with a lid, reduce heat to medium-low, and cook until mushrooms are no longer floating on the surface, about 10 minutes.

STEP 3

Mix tofu and cayenne pepper into miso broth. Tear cooled egg whites into small pieces and add to miso broth. Stir nori and sugar into miso broth; cover pot and simmer, stirring occasionally, until soup flavors have blended, about 1 hour.

Per Serving:

235.2 calories; 13.7 g protein; 29 g carbohydrates; 0 mg cholesterol; 2455.8 mg sodium.

Kid-Friendly Miso Soup

The chicken and the noodles make it more of a meal for the whole family. Skipping the seaweed and the tofu makes it a bit more kid-friendly.

Prep: 10 mins

Cook: 15 mins

Total: 25 mins

Ingredients

1 tablespoon olive oil

½ skinless, boneless chicken breast, diced

4 cups water

1 ½ teaspoons dashi granules

1 (3 ounce) package ramen noodles

cup sliced fresh mushrooms

2 tablespoons chopped green onion

½ cup miso paste

Step 1

Heat olive oil in a skillet over medium heat. Add chicken; cook and stir until no longer pink in the center and the juices run clear, 7 to 10 minutes. Remove to a plate.

Step 2

Bring water to a boil in a medium pot. Add dashi and whisk until granules have dissolved. Reduce heat to medium-low. Add ramen noodles, mushrooms, and cooked chicken; simmer until noodles are tender, about 2 minutes.

STEP 3

While soup is simmering, spoon miso paste into a bowl. Ladle about 1/2 cup of the hot broth into the bowl and whisk with the miso until a smooth paste forms. Add paste to the soup, turn the heat off, and whisk until incorporated. Sprinkle with green onions and serve immediately.

Per Serving:
131.2 calories; 7.6 g protein; 11.2 g carbohydrates; 8.7 mg cholesterol; 1370.9 mg sodium.

Miso Soup I

I am a big fan of miso soup, and this one is fairly straight forward with ingredients that are easy to find. Plus, it tastes great. If you prefer, you can replace the spinach with bok choy.

Prep: 5 mins

Cook: 5 mins

Total: 10 mins

Ingredients

2 ¼ cups water

2 ounces firm tofu, cut into 1/4 inch cubes

1 tablespoon light miso paste

2 teaspoons barley miso paste

½ cup fresh spinach, washed and chopped

1 green onion, thinly sliced

Directions

STEP 1

In a medium saucepan, bring the water to a boil. Ladle out about 1/2 cup of the boiling water, and reserve. Add tofu. Reduce the heat to medium, cover, and cook for 1 to 2 minutes. Add spinach or bok choy; simmer about 1 to 2 minutes, or until the greens are tender. Remove soup from heat.

Step 2

Blend white miso and barley miso into reserved hot water. Stir into soup. Ladle into bowls, and garnish with scallion. Serve immediately.

Per Serving:
48.9 calories; 4.1 g protein; 4.3 g carbohydrates; 0 mg cholesterol; 307.6 mg sodium.

Miso Honey Chicken

It's not hard to make a great marinade with just a few ingredients, as long as one of those ingredients is the magical miso. This super savory paste, made from fermented rice, barley, and soybeans, isn't that hard to find. While the marinade is simple, the flavors are anything but.

Prep: 10 mins

Cook: 45 mins

Additional: 2 hrs

Total: 2 hrs 55 mins

Ingredients
Original recipe yields 8 servings

Ingredient Checklist

3 tablespoons white miso

2 tablespoons honey

¼ cup rice vinegar

2 teaspoons hot sauce

1 tablespoon kosher salt

1 whole chicken, halved, wing tips separated

1 pinch kosher salt to taste

½ lemon, cut into wedges, or to taste

1 pinch cayenne pepper

Directions
Step 1

Combine miso and honey in a bowl. Pour in rice vinegar, followed by hot sauce and salt. Whisk well until mostly smooth. Add chicken halves; cut 3 to 4 slashes into the legs and thighs. Toss chicken in the marinade until well coated. Refrigerate for 2 to 12 hours.

STEP 2

Flip chicken over in the bowl. Sprinkle more kosher salt on top.

STEP 3

Preheat grill to 350 degrees F (175 degrees C) over indirect heat. Add chicken and cover. Grill for 20 minutes and flip chicken over. Cover and grill for another 20 minutes. Brush the excess marinade on top. Cover again and continue cooking until an instant-read thermometer inserted into the center of each thigh reads 165 degrees F (74 degrees C), 5 to 10 minutes more.

Step 4

Plate chicken alongside lemon wedges sprinkled with cayenne pepper. Squeeze some spicy lemon over the chicken as you cut it up.

Tips
Cooking over indirect heat prevents the chicken from burning too much. To achieve this, I used a foil-wrapped ceramic heat diffuser in my grill. If using a regular grill, just place the coals on 1 side and chicken on the other.

Per Serving:

254.6 calories; 26.5 g protein; 6.9 g carbohydrates; 102.5 mg cholesterol; 1119.2 mg sodium.

Homemade Miso Soup
Make your very own Japanese miso soup from scratch. It's

easy to do at home! Perfect for an appetizer or light, warming lunch.

Prep: 10 mins

Cook: 10 mins

Additional: 10 mins

Total: 30 mins

Ingredients

1 tablespoon finely chopped wakame

4 cups water

2 teaspoons dashi granules

3 tablespoons miso paste

4 ounces silken tofu, cubed

2 eaches green onions, sliced on the bias

Directions

Step 1

Place wakame in a fine-mesh sieve and soak in some cold water for 10 minutes.

Step 2

Combine 4 cups water and dashi granules in a saucepan and bring to a boil over medium heat. Add miso paste and whisk to dissolve. Add wakame and simmer for 3 minutes.

Step 3

Divide tofu between 4 serving bowls. Ladle miso soup on top and garnish with green onions.

Per Serving:
46.4 calories; 3.7 g protein; 4.8 g carbohydrates; 0 mg cholesterol; 514 mg sodium.

Chef John's Miso-Glazed Barramundi

This miso-glazed recipe features Barramundi, a mild, flaky, white-fleshed fish that you'll probably be seeing more and more due to its reputation as a sustainable, eco-friendly seafood. It's showing up in grocery store frozen seafood cases, and chances are you'll run across some soon. If you do, buy it and make this recipe.

Prep: 10 mins

Cook: 5 mins

Total: 15 mins

Ingredients

2 tablespoons yellow miso paste

2 tablespoons seasoned rice vinegar

1 tablespoon brown sugar

1 tablespoon soy sauce

2 (5 ounce) barramundi (Asian sea bass) fillets

1 teaspoon vegetable oil

Directions

STEP 1

Whisk miso paste, rice vinegar, brown sugar, and soy sauce together in a bowl until glaze is smooth.

STEP 2

Place barramundi fillets, rounded-side up, onto a plate; spread 1/2 of the glaze onto rounded side of fish.

STEP 3

Heat oil over high heat in a nonstick skillet. Place fish, glazed-side down, in hot skillet and spread remaining glaze over other side; cook until slightly white around the edges, 1 to 2 minutes. Flip fish and cook until flaky and white, 1 to 2 minutes more.

Per Serving:
226.3 calories; 28.5 g protein; 13.3 g carbohydrates; 58.6 mg cholesterol; 1585.9 mg sodium.

Miso Sesame Dressing

Great light dressing to pair with cabbage or romaine lettuce, fresh mandarin oranges, and toasted almonds! Place greens in a bowl and add garnishes. Ladle toasted sesame dressing around salad and toss to coat greens evenly. Sprinkle with 1 teaspoon toasted sesame seeds.

Prep: 5 mins

Total: 5 mins

Ingredients

1 ½ tablespoons miso paste

2 tablespoons rice vinegar

1 ¼ tablespoons honey

1 tablespoon minced fresh ginger root

1 tablespoon sesame oil

1 ½ teaspoons lime juice

1 teaspoon toasted sesame seeds

Directions
Step 1

Whisk miso paste into rice vinegar in a bowl until smooth. Stir honey, ginger, sesame oil, lime juice, and sesame seeds into the vinegar mixture.

Per Serving:

68.9 calories; 0.9 g protein; 7.7 g carbohydrates; 0 mg cholesterol; 242.9 mg sodium.

Miso Soup with Shiitake Mushrooms
A delicious Japanese soup with mushrooms and tofu.

Prep: 10 mins

Cook: 10 mins

Total: 20 mins

Ingredients
4 cups vegetable broth

4 shiitake mushrooms, thinly sliced

¼ cup miso paste

4 teaspoons soy sauce

⅓ cup diced firm tofu

2 eaches green onions, trimmed and thinly sliced

Directions

Step 1

Bring the vegetable broth to a boil in a saucepan. Add the mushrooms, reduce heat to low, and simmer 4 minutes. Stir the miso paste and soy sauce together in a small bowl; add to the broth along with the tofu and continue cooking for 1 minute more. Pour the soup into bowls and top with the green onions to serve.

Per Serving:
91.6 calories; 5.5 g protein; 11.8 g carbohydrates; 0 mg cholesterol; 1405.9 mg sodium.

BBQ Miso Chicken
Boneless chicken marinated in a miso (soy bean paste) sauce and grilled over an open fire. The miso is also mixed with beer, soy sauce, sugar, and sesame oil to give it a complex flavor.

Prep: 15 mins

Cook: 25 mins

Additional: 2 hrs

Total: 2 hrs 40 mins

Ingredients
1 cup miso paste

1 cup beer

1 cup low sodium soy sauce

1 cup white sugar

2 teaspoons sesame oil

⅛ teaspoon cayenne pepper

2 ½ pounds skinless, boneless chicken breast halves

Directions
Step 1

In a large bowl, combine the miso paste, beer, soy sauce, sugar, sesame oil, and cayenne pepper. Stir until the miso and sugar are completely dissolved. Set aside 1/2 cup of the sauce for basting during grilling. Submerge the chicken in the remaining marinade, cover bowl, and refrigerate for at least 2 hours.

Step 2

Preheat grill for medium-high heat.

Step 3

Lightly oil the grill grate. Remove the chicken from the marinade, and discard marinade. Grill chicken for 6 to 8 minutes per side, basting during the last few minutes with the reserved sauce. The chicken is done when its juices run clear.

Per Serving:
484.3 calories; 47.1 g protein; 50.6 g carbohydrates; 107.8 mg cholesterol; 3220.7 mg sodium.

Miso Soup II

This is not a fishy soup like those that are kelp based. Let this soup mellow overnight for best taste. Like all vegetable soups, measures are approximate and substitutions can include whatever vegetable you want. Mushrooms of any kind are particularly good in this soup.

Prep: 25 mins

Cook: 10 mins

Total: 35 mins

Ingredients

2 tablespoons olive oil

¾ cup chopped onion

3 cloves crushed garlic

1 tablespoon minced garlic

½ (12 ounce) package firm tofu, cubed

1 tablespoon soy sauce

1 tablespoon sherry

4 ½ cups water

2 cups grated carrots

1 (10 ounce) package frozen chopped spinach

¼ cup miso paste

ground black pepper to taste

Directions

Step 1

Pour oil into the bottom of a large saucepan, and place

over medium heat. Add onion; saute until tender and almost brown. Add garlic and ginger; saute until fragrant, just a minute or two. Add tofu. Cook, stirring occasionally, until browned; this should take about 5 minutes

Step 2

Stir in soy sauce, thoroughly coating tofu. Add water and sherry. Bring back up to heat, and add carrots and spinach. Heat through.

Step 3

Thin miso with some of the soup, and add back into the soup. Simmer over medium low heat for 5 to 10 minutes, stirring occasionally. Season with black pepper to taste. Serve.

Per Serving:

222.9 calories; 12.7 g protein; 19.7 g carbohydrates; 0 mg cholesterol; 987.2 mg sodium.

Miso Soup I

I am a big fan of miso soup, and this one is fairly straight forward with ingredients that are easy to find. Plus, it tastes great. If you prefer, you can replace the spinach with bok choy.

Prep: 5 mins

Cook: 5 mins

Total: 10 mins

Ingredients

2 ¼ cups water

2 ounces firm tofu, cut into 1/4 inch cubes

1 tablespoon light miso paste

2 teaspoons barley miso paste

½ cup fresh spinach, washed and chopped

1 green onion, thinly sliced

Directions

STEP 1

In a medium saucepan, bring the water to a boil. Ladle out about 1/2 cup of the boiling water, and reserve. Add tofu. Reduce the heat to medium, cover, and cook for 1 to 2 minutes. Add spinach or bok choy; simmer about 1 to 2 minutes, or until the greens are tender. Remove soup from heat.

Step 2

Blend white miso and barley miso into reserved hot water. Stir into soup. Ladle into bowls, and garnish with scallion. Serve immediately.

Per Serving:

48.9 calories; 4.1 g protein; 4.3 g carbohydrates; 0 mg cholesterol; 307.6 mg sodium.

Miso and Soy Chilean Sea Bass
This Sea Bass will melt in your mouth! Delicious, I had this at Blue Water Grill in NYC and it was by far the best sea bass I've ever had in my life. This recipe is as close as I can get to tasting like the restaurants. They served it with bok choy and sticky rice on the side.

Prep: 10 mins

Cook: 7 mins

Additional: 3 hrs

Total: 3 hrs 17 mins

Ingredients

⅓ cup sake

⅓ cup mirin (Japanese sweet rice wine)

3 tablespoons soy sauce

¼ cup packed brown sugar

⅓ cup miso paste

4 (4 ounce) fillets fresh sea bass, about 1 inch thick

2 tablespoons chopped green onion

Directions

Step 1

Whisk together the sake, mirin, soy sauce, brown sugar, and miso paste in a bowl to make the marinade. Place the sea bass in a large sealable plastic bag and pour the marinade over the sea bass. Chill in refrigerator 3 to 6 hours. Arrange the fillets on a baking sheet. Discard the marinade.

STEP 2

Preheat the oven's broiler and set the oven rack about 6 inches from the heat source. Prop the oven door to remain slightly ajar.

Step 3

Bake the sea bass under the broiler until the fish flakes easily with a fork, 7 to 9 minutes. Sprinkle with chopped green onions to serve.

Per Serving:
286.9 calories; 24.7 g protein; 27.9 g carbohydrates; 47.2 mg cholesterol; 1612.5 mg sodium.

Korean Bean Curd (Miso) Soup
This soup is tasty, delicious, easy to make and full of vegetables! This is a very simple Korean soup eaten with rice and other side dishes. Includes tofu, green squash, mushrooms and onions. True Korean recipe! Garnish with sliced green onions.

Prep: 15 mins

Cook: 20 mins

Total: 35 mins

Ingredients
3 ½ cups water

3 tablespoons denjang (Korean bean curd paste)

1 tablespoon garlic paste

½ tablespoon dashi granules

½ tablespoon gochujang (Korean hot pepper paste)

1 zucchini, cubed

1 potato, peeled and cubed

¼ pound fresh mushrooms, quartered

1 onion, chopped

1 (12 ounce) package soft tofu, sliced

Directions
Step 1

In a large saucepan over medium heat, combine water, denjang, garlic paste, dashi and gochujang. Bring to a boil and let boil 2 minutes. Stir in zucchini, potato, mushrooms and onions and let boil 5 to 7 minutes more. Stir in tofu and cook until tofu has expanded and vegetables are tender.

Per Serving:
157.9 calories; 9.1 g protein; 21.6 g carbohydrates; 0 mg cholesterol; 640.7 mg sodium.

Chef John's Miso-Glazed Barramundi
This miso-glazed recipe features Barramundi, a mild, flaky, white-fleshed fish that you'll probably be seeing more and more due to its reputation as a sustainable, eco-friendly seafood. It's showing up in grocery store frozen seafood cases, and chances are you'll run across some soon. If you

do, buy it and make this recipe.

Prep: 10 mins

Cook: 5 mins

Total: 15 mins

Ingredients

2 tablespoons yellow miso paste

2 tablespoons seasoned rice vinegar

1 tablespoon brown sugar

1 tablespoon soy sauce

2 (5 ounce) barramundi (Asian sea bass) fillets

1 teaspoon vegetable oil

Directions

Step 1

Whisk miso paste, rice vinegar, brown sugar, and soy sauce together in a bowl until glaze is smooth.

Step 2

Place barramundi fillets, rounded-side up, onto a plate; spread 1/2 of the glaze onto rounded side of fish.

Step 3

Heat oil over high heat in a nonstick skillet. Place fish, glazed-side down, in hot skillet and spread remaining glaze over other side; cook until slightly white around the edges, 1 to 2 minutes. Flip fish and cook until flaky and white, 1 to 2 minutes more.

Per Serving:

226.3 calories; 28.5 g protein; 13.3 g carbohydrates; 58.6 mg cholesterol; 1585.9 mg sodium.

Miso-Glazed Salmon and Bok Choy

A fast recipe that will have them begging for more! Serve with rice or on a bed of noodles.

Prep: 15 mins

Cook: 10 mins

Additional: 10 mins

Total: 35 mins

Ingredients

½ cup miso

⅓ cup mirin (Japanese sweet rice wine)

¼ cup sake (Japanese rice wine)

3 tablespoons firmly packed brown sugar

2 tablespoons soy sauce

1 ½ pounds salmon fillets

2 heads baby bok choy, halved lengthwise, or more to taste

Directions

Step 1

Stir miso, mirin, sake, brown sugar, and soy sauce in a shallow dish. Add salmon fillets; turn to coat. Marinate at room temperature, 10 to 15 minutes, or in the refrigerator for up to 2 days.

Step 2

Set oven rack about 6 inches from the heat source and

preheat the oven's broiler.

STEP 3

Line a baking sheet with aluminum foil. Transfer fillets onto the baking sheet, reserving marinade.

STEP 4

Place bok choy in the marinade; turn to coat. Arrange bok choy next to salmon on the baking sheet, reserving marinade.

Step 5

Broil in the preheated oven until salmon is lightly charred on the edges, about 4 minutes. Flip salmon and bok choy; brush with reserved marinade. Continue cooking until salmon is browned and flakes easily with a fork, about 3 minutes. Transfer salmon to serving plates. Continue cooking bok choy until it is tender-crisp, 3 to 4 minutes more.

Cook's Notes:

Use yellow or white miso.

Tips

You can also barbeque the salmon, directly on the grill or in a fish basket.

Sesame Tuna with Soy Miso Dressing
This recipe is served at a seafood restaurant in Royal Oak, Michigan. The sesame covered tuna is done medium rare

inside (almost like sushi) and has a fantastic soy miso dressing drizzled over the top. One of the best seafood dishes I love!

Prep: 20 mins

Cook: 4 mins

Total: 24 mins

Ingredients

¾ cup sesame seeds, divided

½ teaspoon seasoning salt

1 teaspoon ground white pepper

1 teaspoon onion powder

1 tablespoon wasabi powder

1 teaspoon coarse kosher salt

1 cup all-purpose flour

2 eggs

3 fluid ounces milk

2 (4 ounce) tuna steaks (about 3/4 inch thick)

2 tablespoons vegetable oil

1 (1.12 ounce) package miso soup mix

1 tablespoon soy sauce

Directions

Step 1

In a shallow bowl, mix together 1/2 cup of sesame seeds, seasoning salt, white pepper, onion powder, wasabi powder, kosher salt and flour; set aside. In a separate bowl, mix together the eggs and milk.

Step 2

Dip tuna steaks in the egg mixture, then dredge in the flour mixture until well coated on both sides. Press on as many extra sesame seeds as possible, so it is well coated. Heat the vegetable oil in a large heavy skillet over medium-high heat. Fry tuna steaks for 2 minutes per side, and immediately remove from heat. The inside of the fish should still be red.

Step 3

To make the soy miso dressing, mix together the miso soup mix and soy sauce. Heat in a small saucepan or microwave, and drizzle over steaks.

Per Serving:

923.7 calories; 52.8 g protein; 71.2 g carbohydrates; 240.1 mg cholesterol; 2377.2 mg sodium.

Japanese Soup with Tofu and Mushrooms

Miso is a fermented soy bean paste that adds a rich flavor. This is a quick, healthy soup that is very popular in Japanese cuisine.

Prep: 10 mins

Cook: 10 mins

Total: 20 mins

Ingredients

3 cups prepared dashi stock

¼ cup sliced shiitake mushrooms

1 tablespoon miso paste

1 tablespoon soy sauce

⅛ cup cubed soft tofu

1 green onion, chopped

Directions

STEP 1

In a medium saucepan, bring stock to a boil; reduce heat to simmer, add mushrooms, and cook for 3 minutes. In a small bowl, mix miso paste and soy sauce together; stir into stock along with tofu. Simmer 5 minutes, and serve topped with green onion.

Per Serving:

100 calories; 11 g protein; 4.8 g carbohydrates; 3.5 mg cholesterol; 1325.8 mg sodium.

Vegetarian Sloppy Joe

My son had one and halfway through the second sandwich he said, 'There's no meat in this!' and finished eating the sandwich. Serve over rice, potatoes, bread, or any other grain.

Prep: 15 mins

Cook: 30 mins

Total: 45 mins

Ingredients

1 tablespoon olive oil

1 small onion, chopped

1 (15 ounce) can brown lentils

1 (15 ounce) can stewed tomatoes, cut small

¼ cup barbeque sauce

¼ cup ketchup

2 tablespoons mild miso paste

1 ounce dried shiitake mushrooms, cut small

2 tablespoons ground allspice

2 cloves garlic, minced, or more to taste

Directions

Heat oil in a large skillet over medium heat. Add onion; cook and stir until soft and browned, about 10 minutes. Add lentils, tomatoes, barbeque sauce, ketchup, miso paste, shiitake mushrooms, allspice, and garlic; cook and stir until flavors combine and mixture thickens, 20 to 25 minutes.

Cook's Note:
Substitute another type of dried mushrooms for the shiitakes if preferred.

Tips
Add hot sauce or ground cayenne pepper to taste.

Per Serving:

231.9 calories; 9.9 g protein; 41.7 g carbohydrates; 0 mg cholesterol; 1023.9 mg sodium.

Hoisin Sauce Home Made

This is a thick, spicy, tangy, sweet, savory Asian sauce, super quick and easy. Perfect as a dipping sauce and marinade. I usually make my own since I have problems with MSG that are normally found in most prepared store-bought sauces. This is a versatile sauce for finger foods and appetizers, for marinating pork, chicken, beef, tofu, and vegetables, as an addition to barbeque sauces, or to complete dishes like mu shu pork, onion pancakes, pot stickers, and dim sum.

Prep: 10 mins

Total: 10 mins

Ingredients
6 tablespoons soy sauce

2 tablespoons seasoned rice vinegar

2 cloves garlic, pressed

2 teaspoons sesame oil

2 teaspoons tahini

1 teaspoon molasses

1 teaspoon apricot jam

⅔ teaspoon brown sugar

⅔ teaspoon miso paste

¼ teaspoon Chinese five-spice powder

⅛ teaspoon red pepper flakes

Directions

Step 1

Place soy sauce, rice vinegar, garlic, sesame oil, tahini, molasses, apricot jam, brown sugar, miso, five-spice powder, and red pepper flakes in a jar with a tight-fitting lid. Seal jar and shake vigorously to combine.

Cook's Notes:

Mix ingredients in a mixing bowl instead of shaking in a jar, if preferred.

Tips

Substitute peanut butter for the tahini, if desired.

Per Serving:

32.9 calories; 1 g protein; 3.8 g carbohydrates; 0 mg cholesterol; 770.4 mg sodium.

Japanese Egg Yolk Sauce

2 Photos

Golden egg yolk sauce similar to what's served in Japanese restaurants. Nice yellow color, firm texture, slightly oily.

Prep: 10 mins

Total: 10 mins

Ingredients

3 eaches egg yolks

½ teaspoon lemon juice

2 ½ tablespoons white miso paste

1 cup vegetable oil

salt to taste

1 pinch freshly ground white pepper

¼ teaspoon grated yuzu (Japanese orange), lemon or lime peel

Directions

STEP 1

In a medium bowl, beat egg yolks and lemon juice with a wooden spoon. Beat in vegetable oil a few drops at a time, beating well after each addition until the mixture begins to emulsify. When all of the oil has been incorporated, stir in the miso, salt, white pepper and grated yuzu. Refrigerate in a squeeze bottle for convenient application.

Quick Sesame Green Beans

This is my interpretation of the green beans from my favorite Japanese restaurant. Serve with a grilled steak! You can omit the miso paste if you choose.

Prep: 10 mins

Cook: 5 mins

Total: 15 mins

Ingredients

8 ounces fresh green beans, trimmed

2 tablespoons low sodium soy sauce

½ tablespoon miso paste

½ teaspoon red pepper flakes

4 cloves garlic, minced

1 teaspoon grated fresh ginger root

1 tablespoon sesame seeds, toasted

Directions

Step 1

Place the green beans into a steamer insert and set in a pot over one inch of water. Bring to a boil, cover and steam for 5 minutes. Remove from the heat and transfer beans to a serving bowl.

Step 2

Meanwhile, in a small bowl, stir together the soy sauce, miso paste, red pepper flakes, garlic and ginger. Pour over the green beans and toss to coat. Sprinkle sesame seeds on top.

Toasting sesame seeds

Heat a dry skillet over medium heat. Add sesame seeds and cook, stirring constantly, until fragrant and lightly toasted.

Per Serving:

45.1 calories; 2.3 g protein; 7.1 g carbohydrates; 0 mg cholesterol; 350.7 mg sodium.

CONCLUSION

When buying miso, choose the unpasteurised, live, enzyme-rich product that will need to be stored in the fridge. This type is loaded with beneficial microorganisms. After opening, the texture, colour and flavour may change so keep an eye on it. Some can be kept for quite a long time without any concerns or variations to quality.

www.ingramcontent.com/pod-product-compliance
Lightning Source LLC
Chambersburg PA
CBHW070314160726
47999CB00003B/1013